# ILEOSTOMY DIET

**The Complete List Of Foods For Ileostomy Patient**

**Discovering Wellness Through Thoughtful Nutrition For Quick Recovery**

**DR. SOFIA SILAS**

# Table of Contents

# CHAPTER ONE

## Introduction

Living with an ileostomy has unique obstacles, but with the right awareness, navigation, and care, people may live happy lives. An ileostomy is a surgical treatment that involves diverting a portion of the small intestine through a hole in the abdomen, resulting in a stoma.

This stoma allows waste to exit without traveling via the colon or rectum. While surgery may be essential to treat illnesses such as inflammatory bowel disease, colon cancer, or trauma, it may have a substantial influence on a person's lifestyle. Individuals, with the correct information and tactics, may adjust to life after surgery while maintaining maximum health and well-being.

## Understanding Ileostomy

An ileostomy significantly modifies how the digestive system works. Instead of going via the colon, waste is ejected straight from the stoma.

This alteration may have an impact on your bowel habits, nutritional absorption, and hydration levels. Individuals with an ileostomy must learn how their digestive system works now and how to deal with possible issues including dehydration, electrolyte imbalances, and skin irritation around the stoma.

Regular follow-up visits with healthcare specialists are essential for monitoring stoma health and resolving any issues that may occur.

## Navigating Life After Surgery

Adjusting to life with an ileostomy requires physical, emotional, and practical concerns. Initially, people may feel anxious, embarrassed, or out of control. It is critical to identify and handle these feelings, and to get help from healthcare experts, support groups, or counselors if necessary. Practical components of post-surgery adaptation include learning how to replace ostomy equipment, regulate odor, and keep the skin surrounding the stoma intact. Individuals may recover confidence and independence in maintaining their ileostomy with time and with practice.

## The Function Of Nutrition In Ileostomy Care

Nutrition is crucial in ileostomy treatment since surgery might impair nutritional absorption and digestion. Certain dietary changes may be required to avoid issues including dehydration, malnutrition, and electrolyte abnormalities. Foods heavy in fiber, spicy, or difficult to digest should be avoided or taken in moderation to reduce the risk of intestinal blockages or discomfort. Maintaining proper hydration is also critical, particularly as patients with an ileostomy may be at a higher risk of fluid loss.

Individuals might benefit from consulting with a certified dietitian to build individualized nutrition regimens based on their unique requirements and preferences.

# CHAPTER TWO

## Creating A Foundation For Wholesome Living

Beyond managing the physical components of ileostomy care, it is critical to prioritize overall health and well-being. This involves remaining physically active, controlling stress, getting enough sleep, and participating in activities that offer pleasure and satisfaction.

Regular exercise not only improves cardiovascular health and muscular strength but also supports proper digestion and bowel function. Stress management practices such as mindfulness, meditation, and deep breathing exercises may help decrease anxiety and enhance general well-being. Prioritizing self-care and establishing realistic objectives may help people live their lives to the fullest, despite the limitations that an ileostomy presents.

## Creating Your Customized Diet Blueprint

Creating a personalized diet blueprint entails testing various meals, evaluating how they influence bowel function and stoma output, and making modifications appropriately.

Individual tolerances and tastes vary, but typical suggestions for an ileostomy diet include eating small, frequent meals and digesting food thoroughly.

Keeping a food journal might help you discover trigger foods and patterns of stomach distress. Gradually reintroducing foods and monitoring their effects may help people extend their dietary options while reducing the chance of issues.

Finally, establishing a balance between eating diverse, healthy food and controlling digestive discomfort is critical to long-term success with an ileostomy.

Living with an ileostomy requires flexibility, knowledge, and proactive self-care. Individuals may successfully manage their condition and live satisfying lives by comprehending the surgical technique, navigating the obstacles of post-operative living, emphasizing good nutrition, supporting general well-being, and developing a tailored nutritional plan.

Individuals with an ileostomy may flourish and pursue their dreams with the help of healthcare experts, peer networks, and personal perseverance.

## Meal Planning Strategies For Success

Meal planning is an essential part of living a healthy lifestyle and meeting nutritional objectives. Individuals who plan their meals ahead of time may guarantee they are eating balanced and healthy foods while also saving time and money.

Effective meal planning includes many critical tactics that help you achieve your health goals.

One of the most important aspects of meal planning is to promote diversity and balance. To achieve optimal nutritional intake, each meal should include a variety of food types.

A well-balanced diet often consists of lean proteins, complex carbs, healthy fats, and an abundance of fruits and vegetables. Individuals may improve the nutritional content and pleasure of their food by integrating a diversity of colors, textures, and tastes.

In addition, portion management is essential for successful meal planning. Portion control is vital for avoiding overeating and maintaining a healthy weight. Using tools like measuring cups, food scales, or visual clues may help people portion their meals appropriately based on their nutritional requirements. Portion management allows people to better regulate their calorie intake and avoid overconsumption, which may contribute to weight gain and other health problems.

Another crucial tip for good meal planning is to prioritize complete, unprocessed foods. Whole foods, such as fruits, vegetables, whole grains, and lean meats, are high in critical nutrients and have no added sweets, harmful fats, or artificial ingredients. Prioritizing these nutrient-dense meals allows people to provide their bodies with the vitamins, minerals, and antioxidants they need for good health. Furthermore, whole meals are often more satiating and may help people feel fuller for longer periods, lowering the risk of excessive snacking and overeating.

Incorporating meal prep into one's routine is also an effective strategy for meal planning. Preparing meals ahead of time may save time on hectic weekdays while also making healthy eating more easy and accessible.

Batch cooking core components like grains, proteins, and veggies help people prepare simple and healthy meals every week. Additionally, portioning meals into containers for quick grab-and-go alternatives might help people avoid the urge to eat unhealthy convenience foods when they are hungry.

# CHAPTER THREE
## Mindful Eating For Optimal Health

Mindful eating is a technique that encourages people to focus on the sensory experience of eating while also raising awareness of hunger signals, emotions, and environmental triggers.

Individuals who practice mindful eating may build a healthy connection with food, improve digestion, and make more conscientious decisions about what and how they eat.

One of the most important aspects of mindful eating is to eat slowly and relish every mouthful. Instead of hurrying through meals, people should chew their food completely, enjoy its tastes and textures, and pay attention to how it makes them feel. Individuals who eat slowly may better detect sensations of satiety and avoid overeating since the body takes time to register fullness.

Another important part of mindful eating is being aware of hunger and fullness signals. Rather than depending on external signals like meal timings or portion levels, people should listen to their bodies and eat when they're hungry, stopping when they're full. Individuals who reconnect with intrinsic hunger and fullness signals might establish a more intuitive eating style and better manage their food intake based on genuine physiological demands.

Practicing mindful eating also entails being aware of emotional and environmental factors that impact eating behaviors. Many individuals resort to food for comfort, stress relief, or diversion, and they often eat it mindlessly in reaction to emotions rather than hunger.

Individuals may build healthy coping strategies and make deliberate choices about how to react to emotional signals other than food by understanding the underlying emotions or events that cause these actions.

Furthermore, mindful eating entails being present throughout the eating experience, from meal planning and preparation to the act of eating itself. This involves being present and engaged throughout meals, without distractions like devices or job duties.

Individuals may increase their enjoyment of their meals and create a deeper appreciation for the sustenance they give by concentrating on the sensory components of eating, such as taste, smell, and texture.

## Nutritional Considerations For Common Challenges.

Navigating common nutritional problems requires a personalized strategy that takes into account individual dietary requirements and preferences. Individuals with food allergies, intolerances, or dietary restrictions may overcome these obstacles by making educated decisions and obtaining help from healthcare experts or trained dietitians.

Individuals with food allergies or intolerances need careful meal planning and label reading to avoid triggering foods and maintain a safe and balanced diet. This might include replacing allergic foods with acceptable substitutes, such as plant-based milks for dairy or gluten-free grains for wheat. Additionally, looking for allergy-friendly recipes and tools may help people broaden their culinary horizons while meeting their nutritional demands.

Dietary limitations, whether owing to cultural, religious, or ethical views, might complicate meal planning. Individuals may, however, discover fulfilling and culturally acceptable nutritional choices by being creative and flexible. Exploring classic foods from many countries, modifying recipes to meet dietary recommendations, and experimenting with new ingredients may all help people maintain a varied and pleasurable diet while following to their limits.

Another typical nutritional concern is weight management and establishing good eating habits. This might include overcoming hurdles like emotional eating, yo-yo dieting, or a lack of nutrition understanding. Individuals may reach and maintain a healthy weight by eating in a balanced and sustainable manner, fueling their bodies with healthful meals. This involves eating nutrient-dense meals, controlling portion sizes, and engaging in regular physical exercise.

## Empowering Yourself With Knowledge

Empowering oneself via information is a key component of effective meal planning and mindful eating. Individuals may make more educated judgments about their health and well-being by educating themselves about nutrition, dietary recommendations, and culinary abilities. This may include looking out for dependable sources of knowledge, such as respected websites, books, or professional organizations, to broaden one's understanding of nutrition and food.

Furthermore, learning practical culinary skills may boost confidence in the kitchen and allow people to produce healthful meals from scratch.

This might involve learning basic culinary methods, knife skills, and recipe adaptations to accommodate personal tastes or dietary limitations. Individuals who learn these core abilities may gain control of their dietary choices and a better feeling of ownership over their health.

Furthermore, getting help from healthcare specialists, such as licensed dietitians or nutritionists, may give tailored advice and encouragement on dietary issues. Working with a skilled expert may provide essential insights and responsibility to help people reach their objectives, whether they are managing chronic diseases, negotiating dietary limitations, or just trying to improve their general health.

In conclusion, meal planning, mindful eating, and nutritional concerns are all essential components of a healthy lifestyle. Individuals may take proactive actions to improve their health and well-being by using strategic meal planning approaches, adopting mindful eating habits, addressing common nutritional issues, and empowering themselves via information.

# CHAPTER FOUR

## Managing Hydration Levels

Hydration is an essential component of general health and well-being, influencing a variety of biological functions and processes. Effective hydration management is knowing the body's water requirements and executing ways to stay hydrated throughout the day.

One of the most important concepts of controlling hydration levels is to drink enough water regularly. The overall suggestion is to drink at least eight 8-ounce glasses of water each day, although individual requirements may vary depending on age, weight, activity level, and environment. Paying attention to thirst signals and getting enough water is critical for avoiding dehydration, which may cause lethargy, headaches, and poor cognitive performance.

In addition to water, electrolytes are essential for staying hydrated, particularly during strenuous physical activity or in hot temperatures.

Electrolytes including sodium, potassium, and magnesium assist manage fluid balance in the body and promote healthy muscular activity. Consuming electrolyte-rich foods and beverages, such as sports drinks or coconut water, may aid in replenishing electrolytes and preventing dehydration after extended activity or exposure to heat.

Monitoring urine color may be a simple measure of hydration level. Light-colored urine normally indicates appropriate hydration, however, dark urine may suggest dehydration and the need for more fluid consumption.

However, it is important to remember that some drugs, supplements, and diets may alter urine color, thus it is not the only indicator of hydration status.

## Exercise And Physical Activity Recommendations

Regular exercise and physical activity are essential components of a healthy lifestyle, with multiple advantages for both physical and mental health.

Participating in a range of activities, such as cardiovascular exercise, strength training, and flexibility exercises, may help improve overall fitness and lower your risk of chronic conditions including heart disease, diabetes, and obesity.

The American Heart Association advises at least 150 minutes of moderate-intensity aerobic exercise or 75 minutes of vigorous-intensity aerobic activity each week, as well as two or more days of muscle-strengthening activities.

Including a variety of aerobic and strength-training workouts in your program may assist enhance cardiovascular health, muscular mass, and metabolism.

In addition to planned exercise sessions, including physical activity in everyday living may improve general health and well-being. Simple modifications, such as using the stairs instead of the elevator, walking or bicycling instead of driving for short excursions, and inserting movement breaks into sedentary pursuits, may assist improve daily activity and aid in weight control efforts.

It is important to listen to your body and choose activities that you love and that are consistent with your fitness objectives. Gradually increasing the intensity and length of exercise sessions may help you avoid injuries and increase your fitness over time.

Consulting with a healthcare practitioner or fitness specialist may give tailored advice based on your specific requirements and fitness level.

## Managing Digestive Issues And Bowel Habits

Digestive health has a substantial impact on overall well-being by influencing nutrition absorption, immunological function, and energy levels. Addressing digestive disorders and keeping regular bowel movements are critical for overall health and quality of life.

Fiber-rich meals including fruits, vegetables, whole grains, and legumes help to promote regular bowel movements and avoid constipation. Aim to include a range of high-fiber foods into your diet to maintain appropriate consumption and promote overall digestive health.

Probiotics, or helpful bacteria that create a healthy gut microbiota, may also aid with digestive health. Yogurt, kefir, sauerkraut, and kimchi are all probiotic-rich foods that may be included in your diet to improve gut health. Furthermore, probiotic pills are available for people who might benefit from greater dosages of beneficial bacteria.

Hydration is another important aspect in ensuring proper digestion. Drinking enough water softens stool and prevents constipation, but dehydration may cause bloating and discomfort. Drink lots of water throughout the day, particularly if you're eating high-fiber meals or doing hard exercise.

# CHAPTER FIVE

## Embracing Emotional Wellbeing

Emotional well-being includes the capacity to handle stress, establish strong relationships, and successfully deal with life's problems. Prioritizing emotional well-being is critical for overall health and resilience, since prolonged stress and unpleasant emotions may cause a variety of physical and mental health problems.

Mindfulness and relaxation strategies may decrease stress and improve emotional well-being.

Meditation, deep breathing techniques, and gradual muscle relaxation may assist in relaxing the mind and body while also improving stress management abilities. Incorporating these activities into your daily routine will boost resilience and general well-being.

Social ties and supportive relationships are equally critical to emotional well-being. Spending time with friends and loved ones, engaging in group activities, and seeking assistance from others during tough times may all help to create a feeling of belonging and emotional resilience. Making an effort to cultivate and maintain strong connections may lead to greater happiness and well-being.

Engaging in enjoyable and fulfilling hobbies may also help to improve emotional well-being. Whether it's pursuing hobbies, spending time in nature, or volunteering in your community, finding things that give your life meaning and purpose will boost your overall happiness and fulfillment.

Taking time for self-care and prioritizing activities that promote emotional well-being is critical for achieving balance and resilience in the face of life's obstacles.

Individuals with an ileostomy have unique obstacles, but with the correct support networks, resources, and methods, they may live happy lives. When helping ileostomy patients, there are several factors to consider, including managing day-to-day activities, navigating social settings, and campaigning for awareness.

# Support Systems And Resources For Ileostomy Patients.

One of the most important aspects of living well with an ileostomy is having access to strong support networks. Support groups, both online and in-person, provide an important chance for patients to interact with people who understand their difficulties directly. These organizations give a forum for exchanging advice, discussing issues, and giving emotional support.

Furthermore, ostomy care specialists play an important role in assisting patients through the first transition phase and providing continuous assistance.

Beyond emotional support, practical tools are critical for ileostomy patients. Access to high-quality ostomy equipment, including as pouching systems and skin care items, is critical for ensuring comfort and preventing problems. Many organizations and charities provide assistance programs to help patients overcome the financial hardship of obtaining these items, ensuring that they have access to the tools they need to survive.

# Travel Tips And Strategies To Live Fully

Traveling with an ileostomy may need more preparation and attention, but it should not prevent people from experiencing the globe and having new experiences. Preparation is essential before starting on a journey, whether it's a quick weekend escape or a longer holiday. Packing an adequate amount of ostomy supplies is critical, since unforeseen delays or changes in routine may occur.

Researching location accessibility and healthcare facilities ahead of time may bring peace of mind and assist in minimizing any issues.

It's also a good idea to notify travel companions or airline personnel about your ileostomy so that you may pass through security checks and use toilet facilities smoothly.

## Adapting To Social Situations: Dining Out

Social events and eating out might be intimidating for ileostomy patients, but with a few tips, they can comfortably manage these circumstances. Open communication with friends, family, and eating businesses is essential for maintaining comfort and meeting any special dietary or bathroom needs.

Choosing restaurants with accessible restrooms and familiarizing oneself with menu selections ahead of time might help reduce anxiety when eating out. It's also a good idea to carry inconspicuous disposal bags for spent ostomy supplies and schedule potty breaks strategically throughout the evening.

## Advocacy And Education To Improve Ileostomy Awareness

Advocacy and education are critical components of raising

awareness and understanding about living with an ileostomy.

There are several fallacies surrounding ostomy surgery, and advocacy activities play an important role in clarifying them and lowering stigma. Individuals may contribute to a more welcoming and inclusive society by sharing their own experiences and increasing awareness about the reality of living with an ileostomy.

Educational programs for healthcare professionals, educators, and the general public are critical for fostering empathy and understanding.

By providing accurate information on ostomy care and addressing common concerns, these initiatives may provide people with the knowledge they need to advocate for themselves and others.

## Conclusion

Living with an ileostomy involves unique obstacles, but with the correct support networks, resources, and methods, people may live full and active lives. Access to support groups, healthcare specialists, and practical tools is critical for negotiating the physical and emotional aspects of living with an ostomy.

By embracing chances for travel, networking, and activism, ileostomy patients may break down barriers, combat misunderstandings, and encourage others to live completely and boldly.

www.ingramcontent.com/pod-product-compliance
Lightning Source LLC
Chambersburg PA
CBHW071004290526
45795CB00005B/1777